PRE-DIABETES COOKBOOK FOR KIDS

Tasty and Nutritious Solutions for Kids' Blood Sugar Control

Dr. Kathrine Williams

COPYRIGHT PAGE

All rights reserved. The copyright holder must provide written permission before any part of this publication can be republished in any manner, such as photocopying, scanning, or other methods.

Copyright ©2024

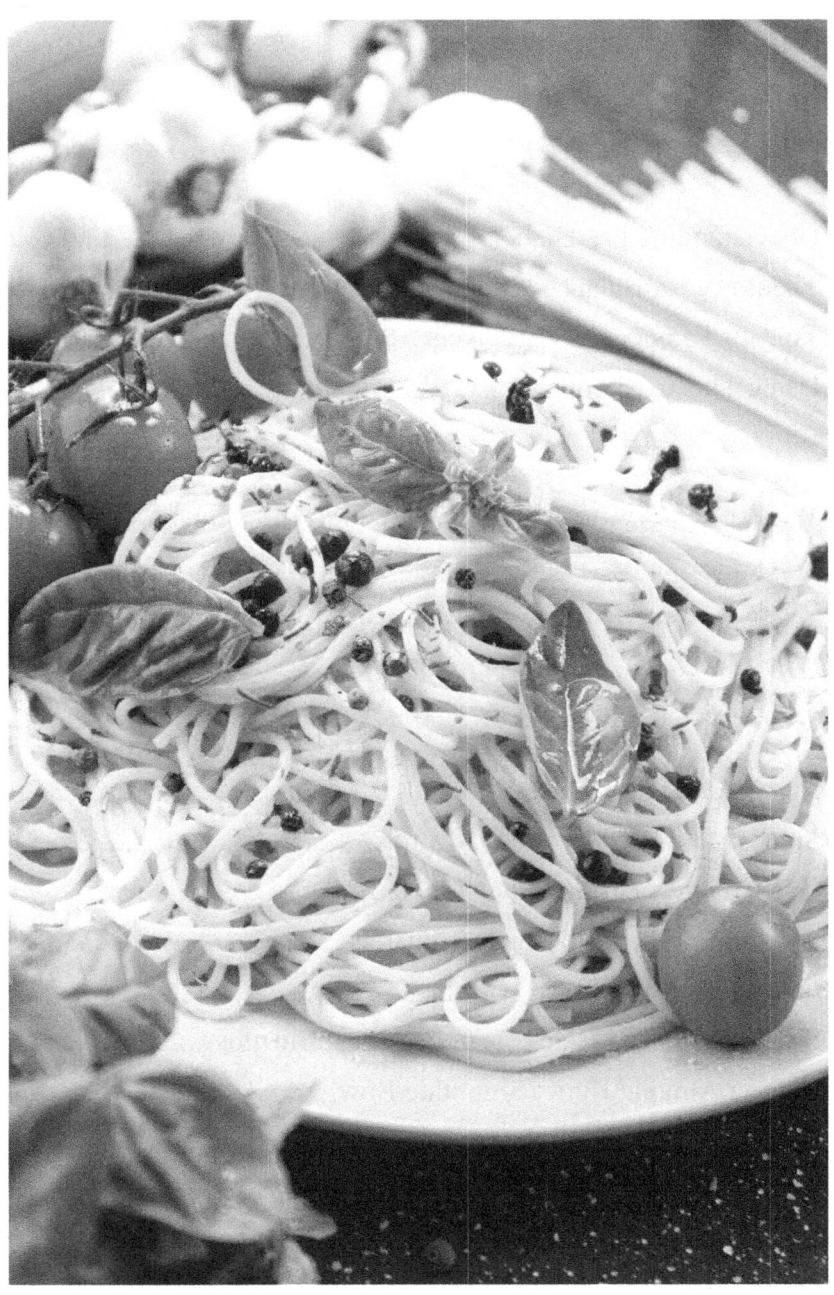

TABLE OF CONTENTS

INTRODUCTION 9

Understanding Pre-Diabetes in Kids 9
The Power of Balanced Meals 9
Tips for Parents and Caregivers 10
Using This Cookbook... 10

Chapter 1: 30-Day Meal Plan 11

Week 1.. 11
Week 2.. 13
Week 3.. 15
Week 4.. 17

Chapter 2: Breakfast Recipes.. 20

Berry Oatmeal Pancakes 20
Spinach and Egg Breakfast Muffins... 21
Greek Yogurt Parfait with Granola 23
Avocado Toast with Cherry Tomatoes.. 24
Quinoa Breakfast Bowl with Fresh Fruit 25
Sweet Potato and Black Bean Breakfast Burritos 26
Banana Almond Butter Smoothie Bowl...................................... 27
Chia Seed Pudding with Berries 28
Scrambled Eggs with Veggies and Whole Wheat Toast................... 29
Apple Cinnamon Overnight Oats.. 30
Healthy Blueberry Muffins 31
Whole Grain Waffles with Fresh Fruit.. 33

Egg and Veggie Breakfast Quesadilla 34
Homemade Breakfast Cereal with Almond Milk 35
Smoothie Bowl with Spinach and Pineapple 36

Chapter 3: Lunch Recipes 38

Turkey and Veggie Wraps 38
Quinoa and Black Bean Salad 39
Chicken and Avocado Salad 40
Sweet Potato and Chickpea Salad 41
Whole Wheat Pasta with Tomato and Basil Sauce 42
Mini Pita Pizzas with Veggies 43
Spinach and Feta Stuffed Chicken Breast 44
Hummus and Veggie Sandwiches 45
Lentil Soup with Carrots and Celery 46
Tuna Salad with Mixed Greens 48
Greek Chicken Pita Pockets 49
Veggie-Stuffed Bell Peppers 50
Chicken and Vegetable Stir-Fry 51
Black Bean and Corn Tacos 52
Veggie Sushi Rolls 53

Chapter 4: Dinner Recipes 55

Baked Salmon with Lemon and Dill 55
Turkey Meatballs with Spaghetti Squash 56
Chicken and Broccoli Stir-Fry 57
Vegetable and Tofu Curry 58
Stuffed Zucchini Boats 60
Beef and Veggie Skewers 61

Sweet and Sour Chicken with Brown Rice 62

Chicken Enchiladas with Whole Wheat Tortillas 63

Mushroom and Spinach Lasagna 64

Baked Cod with Herbs and Lemon 65

Vegetarian Chili with Beans 66

Turkey and Vegetable Shepherd's Pie....................................... 67

Quinoa-Stuffed Bell Peppers.. 69

Cauliflower Fried Rice 70

Lemon Garlic Shrimp with Zucchini Noodles 71

Chapter 5: Snacks and Appetizers 73

Apple Slices with Peanut Butter... 73

Carrot and Celery Sticks with Hummus.................................... 74

Yogurt-Dipped Fruit.. 75

Homemade Trail Mix 76

Whole Grain Crackers with Cheese 76

Baked Sweet Potato Fries... 77

Mini Veggie Frittatas 78

Cucumber Sandwiches with Greek Yogurt Spread.................. 79

Frozen Banana Bites with Dark Chocolate 80

Spinach and Cheese Stuffed Mushrooms................................. 81

Homemade Popcorn 82

Roasted Chickpeas 83

Avocado and Tomato Bruschetta 84

Zucchini Chips 85

Fruit Kabobs 86

Chapter 6: Desserts 88

Frozen Yogurt Berry Bars 88
Baked Apple Slices with Cinnamon 89
Chia Seed Pudding with Mango 90
Dark Chocolate and Almond Energy Balls 91
Peach and Berry Crumble 92
Banana and Oatmeal Cookies 93
Greek Yogurt Chocolate Mousse 94
Apple Cinnamon Muffins... 95
Frozen Banana Pops 96
Sweet Potato Brownies... 97
Berry Sorbet 98
Healthy Pumpkin Pie.. 99
Oatmeal Raisin Cookies 100
No-Bake Energy Bites.. 102
Fruit Salad with Mint 103

Chapter 7: Smoothies 104

Berry Banana Smoothie 104
Spinach and Pineapple Smoothie 105
Mango and Greek Yogurt Smoothie 106
Apple Cinnamon Smoothie 107
Strawberry and Kiwi Smoothie.. 108
Peach and Spinach Smoothie 109
Avocado and Banana Smoothie 110
Green Smoothie with Kale and Pineapple................................ 111
Chocolate Almond Smoothie 112
Orange and Carrot Smoothie 113

Blueberry and Chia Smoothie 114
Tropical Fruit Smoothie 115
Strawberry-Banana Spinach Smoothie................................... 116
Green Apple and Celery Smoothie... 117
Berry and Yogurt Smoothie 118

Conclusion 119

INTRODUCTION

As a parent or caregiver, there's nothing more important than ensuring the health and well-being of your child. But have you ever stopped to consider the long-term risks of unhealthy eating habits? The stark reality is that pre-diabetes in kids is on the rise, and it's up to us to take action.

Understanding Pre-Diabetes in Kids

Pre-diabetes is a condition where blood sugar levels are higher than normal, but not high enough to be classified as type 2 diabetes. It's a warning sign that, if left unchecked, can lead to a lifetime of health complications. The statistics are alarming: according to the Centers for Disease Control and Prevention (CDC), nearly 1 in 5 school-age children in the United States has pre-diabetes.

The Power of Balanced Meals

The good news is that pre-diabetes can often be prevented or reversed through healthy lifestyle choices, particularly when it comes to diet. Balanced meals play a critical role in maintaining healthy blood sugar levels and supporting overall health. By making informed food choices, you can help your child develop healthy habits that will last a lifetime.

Tips for Parents and Caregivers

So, where do you start? Here are some practical tips to get you started:

- Lead by example: Kids often mimic their parents' behavior, so make sure you're modeling healthy eating habits.
- Encourage variety: Expose your child to a wide range of fruits, vegetables, whole grains, and lean proteins.
- Limit processed foods: Try to avoid or limit foods high in added sugars, salt, and unhealthy fats.
- Make mealtime fun: Engage your child in the cooking process and make healthy eating a positive experience.

Using This Cookbook

This cookbook is designed to be a valuable resource in your journey to support your child's health. Inside, you'll find delicious, easy-to-make recipes that are tailored to meet the unique needs of kids with pre-diabetes. With tips, tricks, and expert advice, we'll show you how to make healthy eating a breeze. So, let's get started on this journey together!

Chapter 1: 30-Day Meal Plan

Week 1

Day 1:

- Breakfast: Berry Oatmeal Pancakes

- Lunch: Turkey and Veggie Wraps

- Dinner: Baked Salmon with Lemon and Dill

- Snack: Apple Slices with Peanut Butter

- Dessert: Frozen Yogurt Berry Bars

Day 2:

- Breakfast: Spinach and Egg Breakfast Muffins

- Lunch: Quinoa and Black Bean Salad

- Dinner: Turkey Meatballs with Spaghetti Squash

- Snack: Carrot and Celery Sticks with Hummus

- Dessert: Baked Apple Slices with Cinnamon

Day 3:

- Breakfast: Greek Yogurt Parfait with Granola

- Lunch: Chicken and Avocado Salad

- Dinner: Chicken and Broccoli Stir-Fry

- Snack: Yogurt-Dipped Fruit

- Dessert: Chia Seed Pudding with Mango

Day 4:

- Breakfast: Avocado Toast with Cherry Tomatoes

- Lunch: Sweet Potato and Chickpea Salad

- Dinner: Vegetable and Tofu Curry

- Snack: Homemade Trail Mix

- Dessert: Dark Chocolate and Almond Energy Balls

Day 5:

- Breakfast: Quinoa Breakfast Bowl with Fresh Fruit

- Lunch: Whole Wheat Pasta with Tomato and Basil Sauce

- Dinner: Stuffed Zucchini Boats

- Snack: Whole Grain Crackers with Cheese

- Dessert: Peach and Berry Crumble

Day 6:

- Breakfast: Sweet Potato and Black Bean Breakfast Burritos

- Lunch: Mini Pita Pizzas with Veggies

- Dinner: Beef and Veggie Skewers

- Snack: Baked Sweet Potato Fries

- Dessert: Banana and Oatmeal Cookies

Day 7:

- Breakfast: Banana Almond Butter Smoothie Bowl

- Lunch: Hummus and Veggie Sandwiches

- Dinner: Sweet and Sour Chicken with Brown Rice
- Snack: Mini Veggie Frittatas
- Dessert: Greek Yogurt Chocolate Mousse

Week 2

Day 8:

- Breakfast: Chia Seed Pudding with Berries
- Lunch: Lentil Soup with Carrots and Celery
- Dinner: Chicken Enchiladas with Whole Wheat Tortillas
- Snack: Cucumber Sandwiches with Greek Yogurt Spread
- Dessert: Frozen Banana Pops

Day 9:

- Breakfast: Scrambled Eggs with Veggies and Whole Wheat Toast
- Lunch: Tuna Salad with Mixed Greens
- Dinner: Mushroom and Spinach Lasagna
- Snack: Frozen Banana Bites with Dark Chocolate
- Dessert: Sweet Potato Brownies

Day 10:

- Breakfast: Apple Cinnamon Overnight Oats
- Lunch: Greek Chicken Pita Pockets
- Dinner: Baked Cod with Herbs and Lemon
- Snack: Spinach and Cheese Stuffed Mushrooms

- Dessert: Berry Sorbet

Day 11:
- Breakfast: Healthy Blueberry Muffins
- Lunch: Veggie-Stuffed Bell Peppers
- Dinner: Vegetarian Chili with Beans
- Snack: Homemade Popcorn
- Dessert: Healthy Pumpkin Pie

Day 12:
- Breakfast: Whole Grain Waffles with Fresh Fruit
- Lunch: Chicken and Vegetable Stir-Fry
- Dinner: Turkey and Vegetable Shepherd's Pie
- Snack: Roasted Chickpeas
- Dessert: Oatmeal Raisin Cookies

Day 13:
- Breakfast: Egg and Veggie Breakfast Quesadilla
- Lunch: Black Bean and Corn Tacos
- Dinner: Quinoa-Stuffed Bell Peppers
- Snack: Avocado and Tomato Bruschetta
- Dessert: No-Bake Energy Bites

Day 14:

- Breakfast: Homemade Breakfast Cereal with Almond Milk
- Lunch: Veggie Sushi Rolls
- Dinner: Cauliflower Fried Rice
- Snack: Zucchini Chips
- Dessert: Fruit Salad with Mint

Week 3

Day 15:

- Breakfast: Smoothie Bowl with Spinach and Pineapple
- Lunch: Turkey and Veggie Wraps
- Dinner: Lemon Garlic Shrimp with Zucchini Noodles
- Snack: Apple Slices with Peanut Butter
- Dessert: Frozen Yogurt Berry Bars

Day 16:

- Breakfast: Berry Oatmeal Pancakes
- Lunch: Quinoa and Black Bean Salad
- Dinner: Baked Salmon with Lemon and Dill
- Snack: Carrot and Celery Sticks with Hummus
- Dessert: Baked Apple Slices with Cinnamon

Day 17:

- Breakfast: Spinach and Egg Breakfast Muffins

- Lunch: Chicken and Avocado Salad
- Dinner: Turkey Meatballs with Spaghetti Squash
- Snack: Yogurt-Dipped Fruit
- Dessert: Chia Seed Pudding with Mango

Day 18:
- Breakfast: Greek Yogurt Parfait with Granola
- Lunch: Sweet Potato and Chickpea Salad
- Dinner: Chicken and Broccoli Stir-Fry
- Snack: Homemade Trail Mix
- Dessert: Dark Chocolate and Almond Energy Balls

Day 19:
- Breakfast: Avocado Toast with Cherry Tomatoes
- Lunch: Whole Wheat Pasta with Tomato and Basil Sauce
- Dinner: Vegetable and Tofu Curry
- Snack: Whole Grain Crackers with Cheese
- Dessert: Peach and Berry Crumble

Day 20:
- Breakfast: Quinoa Breakfast Bowl with Fresh Fruit
- Lunch: Mini Pita Pizzas with Veggies
- Dinner: Stuffed Zucchini Boats
- Snack: Baked Sweet Potato Fries

- Dessert: Banana and Oatmeal Cookies

Day 21:
- Breakfast: Sweet Potato and Black Bean Breakfast Burritos
- Lunch: Hummus and Veggie Sandwiches
- Dinner: Beef and Veggie Skewers
- Snack: Mini Veggie Frittatas
- Dessert: Greek Yogurt Chocolate Mousse

Week 4

Day 22:
- Breakfast: Banana Almond Butter Smoothie Bowl
- Lunch: Lentil Soup with Carrots and Celery
- Dinner: Sweet and Sour Chicken with Brown Rice
- Snack: Cucumber Sandwiches with Greek Yogurt Spread
- Dessert: Frozen Banana Pops

Day 23:
- Breakfast: Chia Seed Pudding with Berries
- Lunch: Greek Chicken Pita Pockets
- Dinner: Mushroom and Spinach Lasagna
- Snack: Frozen Banana Bites with Dark Chocolate
- Dessert: Sweet Potato Brownies

Day 24:

- Breakfast: Scrambled Eggs with Veggies and Whole Wheat Toast
- Lunch: Veggie-Stuffed Bell Peppers
- Dinner: Baked Cod with Herbs and Lemon
- Snack: Spinach and Cheese Stuffed Mushrooms
- Dessert: Berry Sorbet

Day 25:

- Breakfast: Apple Cinnamon Overnight Oats
- Lunch: Chicken and Vegetable Stir-Fry
- Dinner: Vegetarian Chili with Beans
- Snack: Homemade Popcorn
- Dessert: Healthy Pumpkin Pie

Day 26:

- Breakfast: Healthy Blueberry Muffins
- Lunch: Black Bean and Corn Tacos
- Dinner: Turkey and Vegetable Shepherd's Pie
- Snack: Roasted Chickpeas
- Dessert: Oatmeal Raisin Cookies

Day 27:

- Breakfast: Whole Grain Waffles with Fresh Fruit
- Lunch: Veggie Sushi Rolls

- Dinner: Quinoa-Stuffed Bell Peppers
- Snack: Avocado and Tomato Bruschetta
- Dessert: No-Bake Energy Bites

Day 28:
- Breakfast: Egg and Veggie Breakfast Quesadilla
- Lunch: Tuna Salad with Mixed Greens
- Dinner: Cauliflower Fried Rice
- Snack: Zucchini Chips
- Dessert: Fruit Salad with Mint

Day 29:
- Breakfast: Homemade Breakfast Cereal with Almond Milk
- Lunch: Sweet Potato and Chickpea Salad
- Dinner: Lemon Garlic Shrimp with Zucchini Noodles
- Snack: Apple Slices with Peanut Butter
- Dessert: Frozen Yogurt Berry Bars

Day 30:
- Breakfast: Smoothie Bowl with Spinach and Pineapple
- Lunch: Turkey and Veggie Wraps
- Dinner: Chicken Enchiladas with Whole Wheat Tortillas
- Snack: Carrot and Celery Sticks with Hummus
- Dessert: Baked Apple Slices with Cinnamon

Chapter 2: Breakfast Recipes

This Chapter of our cookbook, where breakfast becomes both a delightful and nourishing start to your day. These recipes are designed to be flavorful, easy to prepare, and packed with nutrients to keep you energized. Whether you prefer a hearty pancake or a refreshing smoothie bowl, you'll find something to enjoy here. Each recipe is crafted with ingredients that are beneficial for managing blood sugar levels and maintaining overall health.

Berry Oatmeal Pancakes

Ingredients:

- 1 cup rolled oats
- 1/2 cup whole wheat flour
- 1 tsp baking powder
- 1/2 tsp baking soda
- 1/2 tsp cinnamon
- 1/4 tsp salt
- 1 cup almond milk
- 1 egg
- 1 tbsp honey
- 1/2 cup mixed berries (blueberries, raspberries, strawberries)

Instructions:

1. In a large bowl, combine oats, flour, baking powder, baking soda, cinnamon, and salt.

2. In another bowl, whisk together almond milk, egg, and honey.

3. Add wet ingredients to dry ingredients and mix until just combined.

4. Gently fold in berries.

5. Heat a non-stick skillet over medium heat and lightly grease it.

6. Pour batter onto skillet and cook for 2-3 minutes on each side or until golden brown.

7. Serve warm with extra berries if desired.

Nutrition Information (per serving):
- Calories: 250
- Protein: 8g
- Carbohydrates: 38g
- Fat: 6g
- Fiber: 5g
- Sugar: 10g
- Portion Size: 2 pancakes

Spinach and Egg Breakfast Muffins

Ingredients:
- 6 large eggs

- 1 cup fresh spinach, chopped
- 1/2 cup shredded cheddar cheese
- 1/4 cup milk
- 1/4 cup diced bell pepper
- 1/4 cup diced onion
- Salt and pepper to taste

Instructions:
1. Preheat oven to 375°F (190°C) and grease a muffin tin.
2. In a bowl, whisk together eggs and milk.
3. Stir in spinach, cheese, bell pepper, and onion.
4. Season with salt and pepper.
5. Pour mixture into muffin tin, filling each cup about 3/4 full.
6. Bake for 20-25 minutes or until muffins are set and golden.
7. Allow to cool slightly before serving.

Nutrition Information (per muffin):
- Calories: 110
- Protein: 8g
- Carbohydrates: 2g
- Fat: 8g
- Fiber: 1g
- Sugar: 1g
- Portion Size: 1 muffin

Greek Yogurt Parfait with Granola

Ingredients:

- 1 cup Greek yogurt

- 1/4 cup granola

- 1/2 cup mixed berries (strawberries, blueberries, raspberries)

- 1 tbsp honey

Instructions:

1. In a serving glass or bowl, layer Greek yogurt, granola, and berries.
2. Drizzle with honey.
3. Serve immediately or chill until ready to eat.

Nutrition Information (per serving):

- Calories: 280

- Protein: 15g

- Carbohydrates: 35g

- Fat: 8g

- Fiber: 4g

- Sugar: 22g

- Portion Size: 1 parfait

Avocado Toast with Cherry Tomatoes

Ingredients:

- 1 ripe avocado
- 2 slices whole-grain bread
- 1/2 cup cherry tomatoes, halved
- 1 tbsp olive oil
- Salt and pepper to taste
- Optional: red pepper flakes and fresh basil

Instructions:

1. Toast the bread slices until golden.
2. Mash avocado in a bowl and spread evenly over the toast.
3. Top with cherry tomatoes.
4. Drizzle with olive oil and season with salt, pepper, and optional toppings.
5. Serve immediately.

Nutrition Information (per serving):

- Calories: 320
- Protein: 6g
- Carbohydrates: 30g
- Fat: 20g
- Fiber: 9g
- Sugar: 4g

- Portion Size: 1 toast

Quinoa Breakfast Bowl with Fresh Fruit

Ingredients:

- 1/2 cup quinoa, cooked

- 1/2 cup mixed fresh fruit (apple, banana, berries)

- 1 tbsp chia seeds

- 1 tbsp honey

- 1/4 cup almond milk

Instructions:

1. Place cooked quinoa in a bowl.
2. Top with fresh fruit, chia seeds, and honey.
3. Drizzle with almond milk.
4. Mix well before serving.

Nutrition Information (per serving):

- Calories: 280

- Protein: 8g

- Carbohydrates: 45g

- Fat: 8g

- Fiber: 7g

- Sugar: 20g

- Portion Size: 1 bowl

Sweet Potato and Black Bean Breakfast Burritos

Ingredients:

- 1 medium sweet potato, peeled and diced
- 1/2 cup black beans, drained and rinsed
- 1/4 cup diced bell pepper
- 1/4 cup diced onion
- 2 whole-wheat tortillas
- 1/4 cup shredded cheese (optional)
- 1 tbsp olive oil
- Salt and pepper to taste

Instructions:

1. Heat olive oil in a skillet over medium heat.
2. Add sweet potato, bell pepper, and onion. Cook until sweet potato is tender.
3. Stir in black beans and season with salt and pepper.
4. Fill tortillas with sweet potato mixture and top with cheese if using.
5. Roll up and serve warm.

Nutrition Information (per burrito):
- Calories: 320
- Protein: 10g

- Carbohydrates: 50g
- Fat: 10g
- Fiber: 10g
- Sugar: 8g
- Portion Size: 1 burrito

Banana Almond Butter Smoothie Bowl

Ingredients:
- 1 banana, frozen
- 1 tbsp almond butter
- 1/2 cup almond milk
- 1/4 cup granola
- 1/4 cup sliced almonds
- 1/4 cup fresh berries

Instructions:
1. Blend frozen banana, almond butter, and almond milk until smooth.
2. Pour into a bowl and top with granola, sliced almonds, and berries.
3. Serve immediately.

Nutrition Information (per serving):
- Calories: 290

- Protein: 8g
- Carbohydrates: 35g
- Fat: 14g
- Fiber: 6g
- Sugar: 20g
- Portion Size: 1 bowl

Chia Seed Pudding with Berries

Ingredients:

- 3 tbsp chia seeds
- 1 cup almond milk
- 1 tbsp maple syrup
- 1/2 cup mixed berries

Instructions:

1. In a bowl, combine chia seeds, almond milk, and maple syrup.
2. Stir well and let sit for 10 minutes.
3. Stir again, cover, and refrigerate for at least 2 hours or overnight.
4. Top with mixed berries before serving.

Nutrition Information (per serving):
- Calories: 210
- Protein: 6g
- Carbohydrates: 25g

- Fat: 10g
- Fiber: 11g
- Sugar: 10g
- Portion Size: 1 cup

Scrambled Eggs with Veggies and Whole Wheat Toast

Ingredients:

- 2 large eggs
- 1/4 cup milk
- 1/4 cup diced bell pepper
- 1/4 cup diced spinach
- 1 slice whole wheat toast
- 1 tbsp olive oil
- Salt and pepper to taste

Instructions:

1. Heat olive oil in a skillet over medium heat.
2. Add bell pepper and spinach, cook until tender.
3. In a bowl, whisk together eggs and milk.
4. Pour egg mixture into skillet and cook, stirring until scrambled.
5. Serve with whole wheat toast.

Nutrition Information (per serving):

- Calories: 250

- Protein: 12g

- Carbohydrates: 22g

- Fat: 14g

- Fiber: 4g

- Sugar: 4g

- Portion Size: 1 serving

Apple Cinnamon Overnight Oats

Ingredients:

- 1/2 cup rolled oats

- 1/2 cup almond milk

- 1/2 apple, diced

- 1/2 tsp cinnamon

- 1 tbsp honey

Instructions:

1. Combine oats, almond milk, apple, cinnamon, and honey in a jar or bowl.

2. Mix well and refrigerate overnight.

3. Stir before serving.

Nutrition Information (per serving):

- Calories: 220

- Protein: 5g

- Carbohydrates: 35g

- Fat: 6g

- Fiber: 5g

- Sugar: 15g

- Portion Size: 1 serving

Healthy Blueberry Muffins

Ingredients:

- 1 cup whole wheat flour

- 1/2 cup almond flour

- 1/4 cup honey

- 1/2 cup unsweetened applesauce

- 1/2 cup fresh blueberries

- 1/4 cup almond milk

- 1 large egg

- 1 tsp baking powder

- 1/2 tsp vanilla extract

- 1/4 tsp salt

Instructions:

1. Preheat oven to 350°F (175°C) and line a muffin tin with paper liners.
2. In a large bowl, mix whole wheat flour, almond flour, baking powder, and salt.
3. In another bowl, whisk together honey, applesauce, almond milk, egg, and vanilla extract.
4. Combine wet and dry ingredients, then gently fold in blueberries.
5. Divide batter evenly among muffin cups.
6. Bake for 18-20 minutes, or until a toothpick inserted into the center comes out clean.
7. Allow to cool before serving.

Nutrition Information (per muffin):
- Calories: 150
- Protein: 4g
- Carbohydrates: 25g
- Fat: 4g
- Fiber: 3g
- Sugar: 11g
- Portion Size: 1 muffin

Whole Grain Waffles with Fresh Fruit

Ingredients:

- 1 cup whole grain waffle mix
- 1 cup water
- 1 egg
- 1 tbsp vegetable oil
- 1 cup fresh fruit (such as berries, sliced banana, or apple slices)
- 1 tbsp maple syrup (optional)

Instructions:

1. Preheat your waffle iron according to the manufacturer's instructions.
2. In a bowl, combine waffle mix, water, egg, and oil. Stir until smooth.
3. Pour batter onto preheated waffle iron and cook until golden brown.
4. Top with fresh fruit and a drizzle of maple syrup if desired.

Nutrition Information (per serving):

- Calories: 280
- Protein: 7g
- Carbohydrates: 42g
- Fat: 10g
- Fiber: 5g

- Sugar: 12g
- Portion Size: 1 waffle with fruit

Egg and Veggie Breakfast Quesadilla

Ingredients:

- 1 large whole wheat tortilla
- 2 large eggs
- 1/4 cup shredded cheese (cheddar or mozzarella)
- 1/4 cup diced bell peppers
- 1/4 cup chopped spinach
- 1 tbsp olive oil
- Salt and pepper to taste

Instructions:
1. Heat olive oil in a skillet over medium heat.
2. Add bell peppers and spinach, cooking until tender.
3. In a bowl, whisk eggs and pour over veggies in the skillet. Cook until scrambled.
4. Remove egg mixture and set aside.
5. Wipe the skillet and return to heat. Place tortilla in the skillet and sprinkle one half with cheese.
6. Spread egg mixture over cheese, then fold tortilla in half.
7. Cook until cheese is melted and tortilla is golden brown, flipping once.

8. Cut into wedges and serve.

Nutrition Information (per quesadilla):
- Calories: 350
- Protein: 18g
- Carbohydrates: 30g
- Fat: 18g
- Fiber: 5g
- Sugar: 2g
- Portion Size: 1 quesadilla

Homemade Breakfast Cereal with Almond Milk

Ingredients:
- 1 cup rolled oats
- 1/2 cup puffed rice
- 1/4 cup sliced almonds
- 1/4 cup dried fruit (raisins, cranberries)
- 1/4 tsp cinnamon
- 1 cup almond milk

Instructions:

1. In a bowl, combine rolled oats, puffed rice, sliced almonds, dried fruit, and cinnamon.

2. Pour almond milk over the cereal mixture.

3. Stir and let sit for a few minutes before serving.

Nutrition Information (per serving):

- Calories: 230

- Protein: 6g

- Carbohydrates: 35g

- Fat: 8g

- Fiber: 5g

- Sugar: 10g

- Portion Size: 1 cup

Smoothie Bowl with Spinach and Pineapple

Ingredients:

- 1 cup fresh spinach

- 1 cup frozen pineapple chunks

- 1/2 banana

- 1/2 cup Greek yogurt

- 1/4 cup almond milk

- 1 tbsp chia seeds

- 1/4 cup granola

- 1/4 cup fresh fruit (for topping)

Instructions:

1. In a blender, combine spinach, pineapple, banana, Greek yogurt, and almond milk.

2. Blend until smooth.

3. Pour into a bowl and top with chia seeds, granola, and fresh fruit.

4. Serve immediately.

Nutrition Information (per serving):

- Calories: 290
- Protein: 10g
- Carbohydrates: 45g
- Fat: 10g
- Fiber: 7g
- Sugar: 20g
- Portion Size: 1 bowl

Chapter 3: Lunch Recipes

Lunchtime provides an excellent opportunity to enjoy a nutritious and satisfying meal that supports energy levels and overall health. In this chapter, we've gathered 15 lunch recipes that are not only delicious but also crafted with ingredients that help manage pre-diabetes. Each recipe is balanced with proteins, fiber, and healthy fats to keep blood sugar levels steady. Enjoy these wholesome and easy-to-make lunches!

Turkey and Veggie Wraps

Ingredients:
- 1 whole wheat tortilla
- 3 oz. sliced turkey breast
- 1/4 cup shredded lettuce
- 1/4 cup diced bell peppers
- 1/4 cup shredded carrots
- 1 tablespoon hummus
- 1 tablespoon low-fat cheese (optional)

Instructions:
1. Spread hummus evenly over the tortilla.
2. Layer turkey slices, lettuce, bell peppers, and carrots on top.

3. Sprinkle cheese if desired.

4. Roll up the tortilla tightly and slice in half.

Nutrition Information (per serving):

- Calories: 290

- Protein: 20g

- Carbohydrates: 35g

- Fat: 8g

- Fiber: 5g

- Sugar: 5g

- Portion Size: 1 wrap

Quinoa and Black Bean Salad

Ingredients:

- 1 cup cooked quinoa

- 1/2 cup black beans, rinsed and drained

- 1/2 cup corn kernels

- 1/4 cup diced tomatoes

- 1/4 cup chopped red onion

- 1/4 cup chopped cilantro

- 2 tablespoons lime juice

- 1 tablespoon olive oil

- Salt and pepper to taste

Instructions:

1. In a large bowl, combine quinoa, black beans, corn, tomatoes, red onion, and cilantro.

2. In a small bowl, whisk together lime juice, olive oil, salt, and pepper.

3. Pour dressing over salad and toss gently to combine.

Nutrition Information (per serving):

- Calories: 310
- Protein: 12g
- Carbohydrates: 45g
- Fat: 10g
- Fiber: 8g
- Sugar: 6g
- Portion Size: 1 cup

Chicken and Avocado Salad

Ingredients:

- 1 cup cooked, shredded chicken breast
- 1/2 avocado, diced
- 1/4 cup diced cucumber
- 1/4 cup cherry tomatoes, halved
- 1 tablespoon chopped fresh basil
- 1 tablespoon lemon juice

- Salt and pepper to taste

Instructions:

1. In a bowl, combine chicken, avocado, cucumber, tomatoes, and basil.
2. Drizzle with lemon juice and season with salt and pepper.
3. Toss gently and serve.

Nutrition Information (per serving):
- Calories: 280
- Protein: 24g
- Carbohydrates: 10g
- Fat: 18g
- Fiber: 5g
- Sugar: 3g
- Portion Size: 1 serving

Sweet Potato and Chickpea Salad

Ingredients:
- 1 cup roasted sweet potato cubes
- 1/2 cup cooked chickpeas
- 1/4 cup chopped red onion
- 1/4 cup chopped parsley
- 2 tablespoons tahini

- 1 tablespoon lemon juice
- Salt and pepper to taste

Instructions:

1. In a bowl, mix sweet potatoes, chickpeas, red onion, and parsley.
2. In a small bowl, whisk together tahini, lemon juice, salt, and pepper.
3. Drizzle dressing over salad and toss to combine.

Nutrition Information (per serving):
- Calories: 320
- Protein: 10g
- Carbohydrates: 45g
- Fat: 12g
- Fiber: 8g
- Sugar: 9g
- Portion Size: 1 cup

Whole Wheat Pasta with Tomato and Basil Sauce

Ingredients:
- 1 cup whole wheat pasta
- 1/2 cup tomato sauce
- 1/4 cup chopped fresh basil

- 1 tablespoon olive oil

- 1 clove garlic, minced

- Salt and pepper to taste

Instructions:

1. Cook pasta according to package instructions.
2. In a pan, heat olive oil and sauté garlic until fragrant.
3. Add tomato sauce, basil, salt, and pepper.
4. Simmer for 5 minutes.
5. Toss pasta with sauce and serve.

Nutrition Information (per serving):

- Calories: 320
- Protein: 10g
- Carbohydrates: 50g
- Fat: 10g
- Fiber: 7g
- Sugar: 8g
- Portion Size: 1 cup

Mini Pita Pizzas with Veggies

Ingredients:

- 2 mini whole wheat pita breads
- 1/4 cup tomato sauce

- 1/2 cup shredded mozzarella cheese

- 1/4 cup diced bell peppers

- 1/4 cup sliced mushrooms

- 1/4 cup spinach leaves

Instructions:
1. Preheat oven to 375°F (190°C).
2. Spread tomato sauce over each pita.
3. Top with cheese, bell peppers, mushrooms, and spinach.
4. Bake for 10 minutes or until cheese is melted.

Nutrition Information (per serving):

- Calories: 260

- Protein: 12g

- Carbohydrates: 30g

- Fat: 10g

- Fiber: 4g

- Sugar: 5g

- Portion Size: 2 mini pizzas

Spinach and Feta Stuffed Chicken Breast

Ingredients:

- 2 boneless, skinless chicken breasts

- 1/2 cup chopped spinach

- 1/4 cup crumbled feta cheese
- 1 tablespoon olive oil
- 1 clove garlic, minced
- Salt and pepper to taste

Instructions:
1. Preheat oven to 375°F (190°C).
2. Mix spinach, feta, and garlic in a bowl.
3. Stuff chicken breasts with spinach mixture.
4. Brush with olive oil and season with salt and pepper.
5. Bake for 25-30 minutes or until cooked through.

Nutrition Information (per serving):
- Calories: 320
- Protein: 35g
- Carbohydrates: 3g
- Fat: 18g
- Fiber: 1g
- Sugar: 1g
- Portion Size: 1 chicken breast

Hummus and Veggie Sandwiches

Ingredients:
- 2 slices whole grain bread

- 3 tablespoons hummus

- 1/4 cup shredded lettuce

- 1/4 cup sliced cucumbers

- 1/4 cup sliced bell peppers

- 1/4 cup grated carrots

Instructions:

1. Spread hummus on both slices of bread.

2. Layer lettuce, cucumbers, bell peppers, and carrots.

3. Close the sandwich and cut in half.

Nutrition Information (per serving):

- Calories: 280

- Protein: 10g

- Carbohydrates: 35g

- Fat: 12g

- Fiber: 6g

- Sugar: 5g

- Portion Size: 1 sandwich

Lentil Soup with Carrots and Celery

Ingredients:

- 1 cup cooked lentils

- 1/2 cup diced carrots

- 1/2 cup diced celery
- 1/4 cup chopped onion
- 2 cups vegetable broth
- 1 tablespoon olive oil
- 1 teaspoon cumin
- Salt and pepper to taste

Instructions:

1. In a pot, heat olive oil and sauté onions, carrots, and celery until tender.
2. Add lentils, vegetable broth, cumin, salt, and pepper.
3. Simmer for 20 minutes, then serve.

Nutrition Information (per serving):
- Calories: 250
- Protein: 15g
- Carbohydrates: 35g
- Fat: 6g
- Fiber: 10g
- Sugar: 7g
- Portion Size: 1 cup

Tuna Salad with Mixed Greens

Ingredients:

- 1 can tuna, drained
- 2 cups mixed greens
- 1/4 cup cherry tomatoes, halved
- 1/4 cup diced cucumbers
- 1 tablespoon olive oil
- 1 tablespoon lemon juice
- Salt and pepper to taste

Instructions:

1. In a bowl, combine tuna, mixed greens, tomatoes, and cucumbers.
2. Drizzle with olive oil and lemon juice.
3. Season with salt and pepper, then toss gently.

Nutrition Information (per serving):

- Calories: 290
- Protein: 25g
- Carbohydrates: 10g
- Fat: 18g
- Fiber: 4g
- Sugar: 3g
- Portion Size: 1 serving

Greek Chicken Pita Pockets

Ingredients:

- 2 whole wheat pita pockets
- 1 cup cooked, diced chicken breast
- 1/4 cup chopped cucumber
- 1/4 cup chopped tomatoes
- 1/4 cup crumbled feta cheese
- 2 tablespoons Greek yogurt
- 1 tablespoon lemon juice
- 1 tablespoon chopped fresh dill

Instructions:

1. In a bowl, combine chicken, cucumber, tomatoes, feta cheese, Greek yogurt, lemon juice, and dill.
2. Gently mix to combine.
3. Stuff the mixture into pita pockets.

Nutrition Information (per serving):

- Calories: 320
- Protein: 28g
- Carbohydrates: 25g
- Fat: 15g
- Fiber: 5g
- Sugar: 5g

- Portion Size: 1 pita pocket

Veggie-Stuffed Bell Peppers

Ingredients:

- 4 large bell peppers
- 1 cup cooked quinoa
- 1/2 cup black beans, rinsed and drained
- 1/2 cup corn kernels
- 1/2 cup diced tomatoes
- 1/4 cup chopped onions
- 1 teaspoon cumin
- 1/2 cup shredded cheese (optional)
- Salt and pepper to taste

Instructions:
1. Preheat oven to 375°F (190°C).
2. Cut the tops off the bell peppers and remove seeds.
3. In a bowl, mix quinoa, black beans, corn, tomatoes, onions, cumin, salt, and pepper.
4. Stuff the peppers with the mixture and top with cheese if desired.
5. Place in a baking dish and bake for 25-30 minutes.

Nutrition Information (per serving):
- Calories: 280

- Protein: 12g
- Carbohydrates: 40g
- Fat: 8g
- Fiber: 9g
- Sugar: 6g
- Portion Size: 1 stuffed pepper

Chicken and Vegetable Stir-Fry

Ingredients:
- 1 cup cooked chicken breast, sliced
- 1 cup mixed vegetables (broccoli, bell peppers, carrots)
- 2 tablespoons low-sodium soy sauce
- 1 tablespoon olive oil
- 1 clove garlic, minced
- 1 teaspoon grated ginger
- 1 tablespoon sesame seeds (optional)

Instructions:
1. Heat olive oil in a pan over medium heat.
2. Add garlic and ginger, and sauté for 1 minute.
3. Add chicken and vegetables, and stir-fry until vegetables are tender.
4. Stir in soy sauce and cook for another 2 minutes.
5. Sprinkle with sesame seeds before serving.

Nutrition Information (per serving):

- Calories: 290

- Protein: 28g

- Carbohydrates: 15g

- Fat: 12g

- Fiber: 5g

- Sugar: 7g

- Portion Size: 1 cup

Black Bean and Corn Tacos

Ingredients:

- 4 small whole wheat tortillas

- 1/2 cup black beans, rinsed and drained

- 1/2 cup corn kernels

- 1/4 cup diced red onion

- 1/4 cup chopped cilantro

- 1 lime, cut into wedges

- 1 avocado, sliced

Instructions:

1. Warm tortillas in a pan or microwave.

2. In a bowl, combine black beans, corn, red onion, and cilantro.

3. Spoon mixture onto tortillas and top with avocado slices.

4. Squeeze lime wedges over the tacos before serving.

Nutrition Information (per serving):

- Calories: 270

- Protein: 10g

- Carbohydrates: 35g

- Fat: 10g

- Fiber: 8g

- Sugar: 4g

- Portion Size: 2 tacos

Veggie Sushi Rolls

Ingredients:

- 1 cup sushi rice, cooked and cooled

- 4 sheets nori (seaweed)

- 1/4 cup julienned cucumber

- 1/4 cup julienned carrots

- 1/4 cup sliced avocado

- 1 tablespoon rice vinegar

- Soy sauce for dipping

Instructions:

1. Lay a sheet of nori on a bamboo sushi mat or parchment paper.
2. Spread a thin layer of sushi rice over the nori, leaving a 1-inch border at the top.

3. Arrange cucumber, carrots, and avocado in a line across the center of the rice.

4. Roll the nori tightly from the bottom using the mat to help shape it.

5. Slice into bite-sized pieces and serve with soy sauce.

Nutrition Information (per serving):

- Calories: 200
- Protein: 4g
- Carbohydrates: 35g
- Fat: 4g
- Fiber: 4g
- Sugar: 2g
- Portion Size: 6 pieces

Chapter 4: Dinner Recipes

As the sun sets and your day winds down, it's important to enjoy a meal that's not only satisfying but also nutritious. This chapter presents a collection of 15 delicious dinner recipes designed to support your health goals while tantalizing your taste buds. Each recipe balances flavor and nutrition, making it easier to stick to a healthy eating plan.

Baked Salmon with Lemon and Dill

Ingredients:
- 4 salmon fillets (6 oz each)
- 2 tablespoons olive oil
- 2 lemons, sliced
- 2 tablespoons fresh dill, chopped
- Salt and pepper to taste

Instructions:
1. Preheat the oven to 400°F (200°C).
2. Place salmon fillets on a baking sheet lined with parchment paper.
3. Drizzle olive oil over the salmon and season with salt and pepper.
4. Top each fillet with lemon slices and chopped dill.
5. Bake for 15-20 minutes, or until salmon flakes easily with a fork.

Nutrition Information (per serving):

- Calories: 320

- Protein: 28g

- Carbohydrates: 2g

- Fat: 21g

- Fiber: 0g

- Sugar: 1g

- Portion Size: 1 fillet

Turkey Meatballs with Spaghetti Squash

Ingredients:

- 1 medium spaghetti squash

- 1 lb ground turkey

- 1 egg

- 1/4 cup breadcrumbs

- 1/4 cup grated Parmesan cheese

- 1 teaspoon dried oregano

- 1/2 teaspoon garlic powder

- 2 cups marinara sauce

Instructions:

1. Preheat the oven to 375°F (190°C).

2. Cut the spaghetti squash in half and remove seeds. Place cut side down on a baking sheet and bake for 40-45 minutes.

3. In a bowl, combine ground turkey, egg, breadcrumbs, Parmesan, oregano, and garlic powder. Shape into meatballs and place on a baking sheet.

4. Bake meatballs for 25-30 minutes.

5. Scrape cooked spaghetti squash strands with a fork. Top with meatballs and marinara sauce.

Nutrition Information (per serving):

- Calories: 340

- Protein: 30g

- Carbohydrates: 20g

- Fat: 18g

- Fiber: 4g

- Sugar: 6g

- Portion Size: 4 meatballs with 1/2 squash

Chicken and Broccoli Stir-Fry

Ingredients:

- 1 lb chicken breast, sliced

- 2 cups broccoli florets

- 1 tablespoon olive oil

- 1/4 cup low-sodium soy sauce

- 1 tablespoon honey

- 2 cloves garlic, minced

- 1 teaspoon grated ginger

Instructions:

1. Heat olive oil in a large skillet over medium-high heat.

2. Add chicken and cook until no longer pink, about 5-7 minutes.

3. Add garlic and ginger, cooking for 1 more minute.

4. Stir in broccoli and cook until tender-crisp, about 3-4 minutes.

5. Add soy sauce and honey, stirring until well coated. Serve hot.

Nutrition Information (per serving):

- Calories: 290
- Protein: 28g
- Carbohydrates: 15g
- Fat: 13g
- Fiber: 3g
- Sugar: 9g
- Portion Size: 1 cup

Vegetable and Tofu Curry

Ingredients:

- 1 block firm tofu, cubed
- 1 cup bell peppers, chopped
- 1 cup carrots, sliced
- 1 cup cauliflower florets

- 1 can (14 oz) coconut milk
- 2 tablespoons curry powder
- 1 tablespoon olive oil
- Salt to taste

Instructions:
1. Heat olive oil in a large pan over medium heat.
2. Add tofu and cook until golden brown, about 5 minutes. Remove tofu and set aside.
3. In the same pan, add bell peppers, carrots, and cauliflower. Cook for 5 minutes.
4. Stir in curry powder and coconut milk. Simmer for 10 minutes.
5. Return tofu to the pan, stirring until heated through. Serve with rice.

Nutrition Information (per serving):
- Calories: 340
- Protein: 15g
- Carbohydrates: 30g
- Fat: 22g
- Fiber: 6g
- Sugar: 6g
- Portion Size: 1 cup

Stuffed Zucchini Boats

Ingredients:

- 4 medium zucchinis, halved lengthwise

- 1/2 cup cooked quinoa

- 1/2 cup marinara sauce

- 1/2 cup shredded mozzarella cheese

- 1/4 cup grated Parmesan cheese

- 1/2 cup chopped mushrooms

Instructions:

1. Preheat the oven to 375°F (190°C).

2. Scoop out the center of zucchini halves to create boats.

3. In a bowl, mix cooked quinoa, marinara sauce, mushrooms, and half of the mozzarella cheese.

4. Fill zucchini boats with the mixture and top with remaining cheese.

5. Bake for 20-25 minutes until zucchini is tender and cheese is melted.

Nutrition Information (per serving):

- Calories: 210

- Protein: 14g

- Carbohydrates: 20g

- Fat: 10g

- Fiber: 5g
- Sugar: 6g
- Portion Size: 2 boats

Beef and Veggie Skewers

Ingredients:
- 1 lb beef sirloin, cubed
- 1 cup bell peppers, chopped
- 1 cup cherry tomatoes
- 1 cup onions, chopped
- 2 tablespoons olive oil
- 1 tablespoon balsamic vinegar
- Salt and pepper to taste

Instructions:
1. Preheat grill to medium-high heat.
2. Thread beef and vegetables onto skewers.
3. Brush with olive oil and balsamic vinegar, then season with salt and pepper.
4. Grill skewers for 10-15 minutes, turning occasionally, until beef is cooked to desired doneness.

Nutrition Information (per serving):
- Calories: 280

- Protein: 25g

- Carbohydrates: 10g

- Fat: 18g

- Fiber: 3g

- Sugar: 5g

- Portion Size: 3 skewers

Sweet and Sour Chicken with Brown Rice

Ingredients:

- 1 lb chicken breast, cubed

- 1/2 cup pineapple chunks

- 1/4 cup bell pepper, chopped

- 1/4 cup onion, chopped

- 1/4 cup low-sodium soy sauce

- 2 tablespoons honey

- 1 tablespoon rice vinegar

- 1 cup cooked brown rice

Instructions:

1. In a large skillet, cook chicken over medium heat until browned.
2. Add bell pepper, onion, and pineapple, cooking for 5 minutes.
3. Stir in soy sauce, honey, and rice vinegar, simmering until sauce thickens.
4. Serve over brown rice.

Nutrition Information (per serving):

- Calories: 340
- Protein: 28g
- Carbohydrates: 30g
- Fat: 10g
- Fiber: 4g
- Sugar: 12g
- Portion Size: 1 cup with 1/2 cup rice

Chicken Enchiladas with Whole Wheat Tortillas

Ingredients:

- 2 cups shredded chicken
- 1 cup black beans
- 1 cup shredded cheese
- 1 cup enchilada sauce
- 8 whole wheat tortillas

Instructions:

1. Preheat oven to 375°F (190°C).
2. Fill tortillas with chicken, beans, and cheese, then roll up and place in a baking dish.
3. Pour enchilada sauce over tortillas and top with remaining cheese.
4. Bake for 20 minutes, until cheese is melted and bubbly.

Nutrition Information (per serving):

- Calories: 360

- Protein: 28g

- Carbohydrates: 35g

- Fat: 15g

- Fiber: 8g

- Sugar: 6g

- Portion Size: 2 enchiladas

Mushroom and Spinach Lasagna

Ingredients:

- 9 whole wheat lasagna noodles

- 2 cups ricotta cheese

- 1 cup shredded mozzarella cheese

- 2 cups chopped spinach

- 1 cup sliced mushrooms

- 2 cups marinara sauce

Instructions:

1. Preheat oven to 375°F (190°C).

2. Cook lasagna noodles according to package instructions.

3. In a baking dish, layer noodles, ricotta cheese, spinach, mushrooms, and marinara sauce.

4. Top with mozzarella cheese and bake for 30 minutes.

Nutrition Information (per serving):

- Calories: 350

- Protein: 20g

- Carbohydrates: 35g

- Fat: 15g

- Fiber: 4g

- Sugar: 8g

- Portion Size: 1 slice

Baked Cod with Herbs and Lemon

Ingredients:

- 4 cod fillets (6 oz each)

- 2 tablespoons olive oil

- 1 lemon, sliced

- 1 tablespoon fresh thyme, chopped

- Salt and pepper to taste

Instructions:

1. Preheat the oven to 375°F (190°C).
2. Place cod fillets on a baking sheet lined with parchment paper.
3. Drizzle with olive oil and season with salt and pepper.
4. Top with lemon slices and sprinkle with fresh thyme.
5. Bake for 15-20 minutes, or until the fish flakes easily with a fork.

Nutrition Information (per serving):

- Calories: 250

- Protein: 30g

- Carbohydrates: 1g

- Fat: 14g

- Fiber: 0g

- Sugar: 1g

- Portion Size: 1 fillet

Vegetarian Chili with Beans

Ingredients:

- 1 tablespoon olive oil

- 1 onion, chopped

- 2 cloves garlic, minced

- 1 bell pepper, chopped

- 1 cup carrots, diced

- 1 can (14 oz) diced tomatoes

- 1 can (14 oz) kidney beans, drained

- 1 can (14 oz) black beans, drained

- 1 cup corn kernels

- 2 tablespoons chili powder

- 1 teaspoon cumin

- Salt and pepper to taste

Instructions:

1. Heat olive oil in a large pot over medium heat.

2. Add onion and garlic, cooking until softened, about 5 minutes.

3. Add bell pepper and carrots, cooking for another 5 minutes.

4. Stir in diced tomatoes, kidney beans, black beans, corn, chili powder, cumin, salt, and pepper.

5. Simmer for 20-25 minutes, stirring occasionally.

Nutrition Information (per serving):

- Calories: 280
- Protein: 15g
- Carbohydrates: 45g
- Fat: 5g
- Fiber: 12g
- Sugar: 8g
- Portion Size: 1 cup

Turkey and Vegetable Shepherd's Pie

Ingredients:

- 1 lb ground turkey
- 1 cup carrots, diced
- 1 cup peas
- 1 cup corn kernels
- 1/2 cup onion, chopped

- 2 cloves garlic, minced
- 1/2 cup chicken broth
- 2 tablespoons flour
- 1/2 teaspoon dried thyme
- 2 cups mashed sweet potatoes

Instructions:
1. Preheat oven to 375°F (190°C).
2. In a skillet, cook ground turkey until browned. Remove and set aside.
3. In the same skillet, cook onions and garlic until softened. Add carrots, peas, and corn, cooking until tender.
4. Stir in flour, cook for 1 minute, then add chicken broth and thyme, simmering until thickened.
5. Return turkey to the skillet and mix well.
6. Transfer mixture to a baking dish and top with mashed sweet potatoes.
7. Bake for 20 minutes, until the top is golden brown.

Nutrition Information (per serving):
- Calories: 350
- Protein: 30g
- Carbohydrates: 40g
- Fat: 10g

- Fiber: 7g
- Sugar: 9g
- Portion Size: 1 cup

Quinoa-Stuffed Bell Peppers

Ingredients:
- 4 bell peppers, tops cut off and seeds removed
- 1 cup cooked quinoa
- 1/2 cup black beans, drained
- 1/2 cup corn kernels
- 1/2 cup diced tomatoes
- 1/4 cup shredded cheese (optional)
- 1 teaspoon cumin
- 1/2 teaspoon paprika
- Salt and pepper to taste

Instructions:
1. Preheat oven to 375°F (190°C).
2. In a bowl, mix quinoa, black beans, corn, tomatoes, cumin, paprika, salt, and pepper.
3. Stuff each bell pepper with the quinoa mixture.
4. Place peppers in a baking dish and top with cheese if using.
5. Bake for 25-30 minutes, until peppers are tender.

Nutrition Information (per serving):

- Calories: 280
- Protein: 12g
- Carbohydrates: 45g
- Fat: 8g
- Fiber: 8g
- Sugar: 7g
- Portion Size: 1 stuffed pepper

Cauliflower Fried Rice

Ingredients:

- 1 head cauliflower, grated into rice-sized pieces
- 1 tablespoon olive oil
- 1 cup mixed vegetables (carrots, peas, corn)
- 2 eggs, lightly beaten
- 2 cloves garlic, minced
- 2 tablespoons soy sauce
- 1 green onion, chopped

Instructions:

1. Heat olive oil in a large skillet over medium heat.
2. Add garlic and cook for 1 minute.
3. Add mixed vegetables and cook until tender.

4. Push vegetables to one side of the skillet and pour eggs into the other side. Scramble eggs until cooked through.

5. Add cauliflower rice and soy sauce, stirring to combine. Cook for 5-7 minutes, until cauliflower is tender.

6. Garnish with green onions before serving.

Nutrition Information (per serving):
- Calories: 210
- Protein: 10g
- Carbohydrates: 20g
- Fat: 12g
- Fiber: 5g
- Sugar: 5g
- Portion Size: 1 cup

Lemon Garlic Shrimp with Zucchini Noodles

Ingredients:
- 1 lb large shrimp, peeled and deveined
- 2 tablespoons olive oil
- 4 cloves garlic, minced
- 1 tablespoon lemon juice
- 1 teaspoon lemon zest
- 4 cups zucchini noodles

- Salt and pepper to taste

Instructions:

1. Heat olive oil in a skillet over medium-high heat.

2. Add garlic and cook for 1 minute.

3. Add shrimp and cook for 3-4 minutes per side, until pink and opaque.

4. Stir in lemon juice and zest, then add zucchini noodles.

5. Cook for an additional 2-3 minutes, until zucchini is tender.

Nutrition Information (per serving):

- Calories: 250
- Protein: 25g
- Carbohydrates: 10g
- Fat: 12g
- Fiber: 3g
- Sugar: 5g
- Portion Size: 1 cup

Chapter 5: Snacks and Appetizers

Snacks and appetizers can play a vital role in maintaining a healthy diet, especially when managing pre-diabetes. Choosing nutritious, satisfying options can help stabilize blood sugar levels and curb hunger between meals. This chapter presents a selection of snacks and appetizers that are not only delicious but also align with dietary needs. Here's a collection of recipes that offer balanced flavors and nutrients to keep you energized and satisfied.

Apple Slices with Peanut Butter

Ingredients:

- 2 medium apples, cored and sliced
- 2 tablespoons peanut butter (natural, no sugar added)

Instructions:

1. Wash and core the apples, then slice them into thin rounds.
2. Spread a thin layer of peanut butter over each apple slice.
3. Serve immediately or refrigerate for a quick snack.

Nutrition Information (per serving):
- Calories: 150
- Protein: 4g

- Carbohydrates: 22g
- Fat: 7g
- Fiber: 4g
- Sugar: 15g
- Portion Size: 1 apple with 2 tablespoons of peanut butter

Carrot and Celery Sticks with Hummus

Ingredients:
- 1 cup baby carrots
- 1 cup celery sticks
- 1/2 cup hummus

Instructions:
1. Wash and cut the carrots and celery into sticks.
2. Arrange the vegetable sticks on a plate.
3. Serve with a side of hummus for dipping.

Nutrition Information (per serving):
- Calories: 120
- Protein: 4g
- Carbohydrates: 20g
- Fat: 4g
- Fiber: 5g
- Sugar: 8g

- Portion Size: 1 cup of vegetables with 1/4 cup hummus

Yogurt-Dipped Fruit

Ingredients:

- 1 cup strawberries, hulled
- 1 cup blueberries
- 1 cup plain Greek yogurt
- 1 tablespoon honey (optional)

Instructions:

1. Wash and prepare the fruit.
2. In a bowl, mix Greek yogurt with honey, if using.
3. Dip the fruit into the yogurt and enjoy.

Nutrition Information (per serving):

- Calories: 110
- Protein: 6g
- Carbohydrates: 22g
- Fat: 1g
- Fiber: 3g
- Sugar: 17g
- Portion Size: 1 cup of fruit with 1/2 cup yogurt

Homemade Trail Mix

Ingredients:

- 1/2 cup almonds
- 1/2 cup walnuts
- 1/4 cup dried cranberries
- 1/4 cup dark chocolate chips
- 1/4 cup pumpkin seeds

Instructions:

1. Mix all ingredients in a bowl.
2. Store in an airtight container for a convenient snack.

Nutrition Information (per serving):

- Calories: 200
- Protein: 6g
- Carbohydrates: 18g
- Fat: 14g
- Fiber: 3g
- Sugar: 12g
- Portion Size: 1/4 cup

Whole Grain Crackers with Cheese

Ingredients:

- 6 whole grain crackers

- 2 ounces low-fat cheese, sliced

Instructions:
1. Arrange crackers on a plate.
2. Top each cracker with a slice of cheese.
3. Serve immediately.

Nutrition Information (per serving):
- Calories: 180
- Protein: 8g
- Carbohydrates: 22g
- Fat: 8g
- Fiber: 4g
- Sugar: 2g
- Portion Size: 6 crackers with 2 ounces of cheese

Baked Sweet Potato Fries

Ingredients:
- 2 medium sweet potatoes, peeled and cut into fries
- 1 tablespoon olive oil
- 1 teaspoon paprika
- Salt and pepper to taste

Instructions:

1. Preheat the oven to 425°F (220°C).

2. Toss sweet potato fries with olive oil, paprika, salt, and pepper.

3. Spread on a baking sheet in a single layer.

4. Bake for 20-25 minutes or until crispy.

Nutrition Information (per serving):

- Calories: 150

- Protein: 2g

- Carbohydrates: 30g

- Fat: 5g

- Fiber: 4g

- Sugar: 7g

- Portion Size: 1 cup

Mini Veggie Frittatas

Ingredients:

- 6 large eggs

- 1 cup chopped spinach

- 1/2 cup diced bell peppers

- 1/4 cup shredded cheese

- Salt and pepper to taste

Instructions:

1. Preheat the oven to 375°F (190°C).

2. Whisk eggs in a bowl, then stir in spinach, bell peppers, cheese, salt, and pepper.

3. Pour mixture into a greased muffin tin.

4. Bake for 15-20 minutes or until set.

Nutrition Information (per serving):

- Calories: 120
- Protein: 8g
- Carbohydrates: 3g
- Fat: 9g
- Fiber: 1g
- Sugar: 2g
- Portion Size: 1 mini frittata

Cucumber Sandwiches with Greek Yogurt Spread

Ingredients:

- 1 cucumber, thinly sliced
- 4 whole grain sandwich slices
- 1/2 cup Greek yogurt
- 1 tablespoon fresh dill, chopped
- Salt and pepper to taste

Instructions:

1. Mix Greek yogurt with dill, salt, and pepper.

2. Spread the mixture on one side of each bread slice.

3. Layer cucumber slices on half of the bread slices.

4. Top with the remaining bread slices and cut into quarters.

Nutrition Information (per serving):

- Calories: 140

- Protein: 6g

- Carbohydrates: 20g

- Fat: 5g

- Fiber: 3g

- Sugar: 4g

- Portion Size: 2 sandwich quarters

Frozen Banana Bites with Dark Chocolate

Ingredients:

- 2 ripe bananas, sliced

- 1/2 cup dark chocolate chips

- 1 tablespoon coconut oil

Instructions:

1. Melt chocolate chips and coconut oil in a microwave-safe bowl.

2. Dip banana slices into the melted chocolate.

3. Place on a baking sheet lined with parchment paper.

4. Freeze until solid.

Nutrition Information (per serving):

- Calories: 150

- Protein: 2g

- Carbohydrates: 21g

- Fat: 7g

- Fiber: 2g

- Sugar: 14g

- Portion Size: 4-5 bites

Spinach and Cheese Stuffed Mushrooms

Ingredients:

- 12 large mushrooms, stems removed

- 1 cup chopped spinach

- 1/2 cup shredded cheese

- 1 clove garlic, minced

- 1 tablespoon olive oil

Instructions:

1. Preheat the oven to 375°F (190°C).

2. Mix spinach, cheese, garlic, and olive oil in a bowl.

3. Stuff each mushroom cap with the mixture.

4. Bake for 15-20 minutes until tender.

Nutrition Information (per serving):

- Calories: 100
- Protein: 6g
- Carbohydrates: 5g
- Fat: 7g
- Fiber: 2g
- Sugar: 2g
- Portion Size: 4 mushrooms

Homemade Popcorn

Ingredients:

- 1/2 cup popcorn kernels
- 1 tablespoon olive oil
- Salt to taste

Instructions:

1. Heat olive oil in a large pot over medium heat.
2. Add popcorn kernels and cover the pot.
3. Shake the pot occasionally until popping slows.
4. Remove from heat and season with salt.

Nutrition Information (per serving):

- Calories: 130
- Protein: 3g
- Carbohydrates: 24g
- Fat: 3g
- Fiber: 4g
- Sugar: 0g
- Portion Size: 3 cups popped popcorn

Roasted Chickpeas

Ingredients:

- 1 can chickpeas, drained and rinsed
- 1 tablespoon olive oil
- 1 teaspoon paprika
- Salt to taste

Instructions:
1. Preheat the oven to 400°F (200°C).
2. Toss chickpeas with olive oil, paprika, and salt.
3. Spread on a baking sheet and roast for 20-30 minutes until crispy.

Nutrition Information (per serving):

- Calories: 150
- Protein: 6g

- Carbohydrates: 20g
- Fat: 6g
- Fiber: 5g
- Sugar: 3g
- Portion Size: 1/2 cup

Avocado and Tomato Bruschetta

Ingredients:
- 1 avocado, diced
- 1 cup cherry tomatoes, halved
- 1 tablespoon olive oil
- 1 tablespoon fresh basil, chopped
- Salt and pepper to taste
- 6 slices whole grain baguette, toasted

Instructions:
1. Mix avocado, tomatoes, olive oil, basil, salt, and pepper in a bowl.
2. Spoon mixture onto toasted baguette slices.
3. Serve immediately.

Nutrition Information (per serving):
- Calories: 180
- Protein: 4g
- Carbohydrates: 22g

- Fat: 10g
- Fiber: 6g
- Sugar: 4g
- Portion Size: 2 slices of bruschetta

Zucchini Chips

Ingredients:
- 2 medium zucchinis, thinly sliced
- 1 tablespoon olive oil
- 1/2 teaspoon garlic powder
- 1/2 teaspoon onion powder
- Salt to taste

Instructions:
1. Preheat the oven to 425°F (220°C).
2. Toss zucchini slices with olive oil, garlic powder, onion powder, and salt.
3. Arrange slices in a single layer on a baking sheet.
4. Bake for 15-20 minutes or until crispy, flipping halfway through.

Nutrition Information (per serving):
- Calories: 100
- Protein: 2g
- Carbohydrates: 10g

- Fat: 6g
- Fiber: 3g
- Sugar: 3g
- Portion Size: 1 cup

Fruit Kabobs

Ingredients:
- 1 cup strawberries, hulled
- 1 cup pineapple chunks
- 1 cup grapes
- 1 cup melon cubes
- Wooden skewers

Instructions:
1. Thread strawberries, pineapple chunks, grapes, and melon cubes onto wooden skewers.
2. Arrange the kabobs on a plate and serve.

Nutrition Information (per serving):
- Calories: 80
- Protein: 1g
- Carbohydrates: 21g
- Fat: 0g
- Fiber: 2g

- Sugar: 16g
- Portion Size: 2 kabobs

Chapter 6: Desserts

Desserts can be a delightful end to any meal, and when you're managing pre-diabetes, choosing the right ones is essential. This chapter features a variety of healthy, indulgent desserts that satisfy your sweet tooth while keeping your blood sugar in check. From fruity sorbets to rich chocolate treats, each recipe is designed to offer a balance of taste and nutrition.

Frozen Yogurt Berry Bars

Ingredients:

- 2 cups mixed berries (strawberries, blueberries, raspberries)
- 1 cup plain Greek yogurt
- 2 tablespoons honey
- 1 teaspoon vanilla extract

Instructions:

1. Puree the berries in a blender or food processor until smooth.
2. In a bowl, mix the Greek yogurt, honey, and vanilla extract.
3. Stir the berry puree into the yogurt mixture until well combined.
4. Pour the mixture into a baking dish lined with parchment paper.
5. Freeze for at least 4 hours or until solid.
6. Cut into bars and serve.

Nutrition Information (per bar, based on 8 servings):

- Calories: 120
- Protein: 5g
- Carbohydrates: 18g
- Fat: 2g
- Fiber: 3g
- Sugar: 14g
- Portion Size: 1 bar

Baked Apple Slices with Cinnamon

Ingredients:

- 4 medium apples, cored and sliced
- 2 tablespoons cinnamon
- 1 tablespoon honey
- 1/2 teaspoon nutmeg

Instructions:

1. Preheat your oven to 350°F (175°C).
2. Arrange apple slices on a baking sheet in a single layer.
3. Drizzle honey over the apples and sprinkle with cinnamon and nutmeg.
4. Bake for 20-25 minutes, or until apples are tender and slightly caramelized.
5. Serve warm or at room temperature.

Nutrition Information (per serving, based on 4 servings):

- Calories: 100

- Protein: 0g

- Carbohydrates: 27g

- Fat: 0g

- Fiber: 4g

- Sugar: 22g

- Portion Size: 1/4 of recipe

Chia Seed Pudding with Mango

Ingredients:

- 1/4 cup chia seeds

- 1 cup almond milk

- 1 tablespoon honey

- 1 ripe mango, peeled and diced

Instructions:

1. In a bowl, combine chia seeds, almond milk, and honey.

2. Stir well and let sit for 10 minutes, then stir again.

3. Cover and refrigerate for at least 4 hours or overnight.

4. Before serving, top with diced mango.

Nutrition Information (per serving, based on 2 servings):

- Calories: 180

- Protein: 4g
- Carbohydrates: 30g
- Fat: 7g
- Fiber: 10g
- Sugar: 17g
- Portion Size: 1/2 of recipe

Dark Chocolate and Almond Energy Balls

Ingredients:
- 1 cup almonds
- 1 cup dates, pitted
- 1/4 cup unsweetened cocoa powder
- 1 tablespoon honey

Instructions:
1. In a food processor, blend almonds until finely chopped.
2. Add dates, cocoa powder, and honey. Blend until the mixture forms a sticky dough.
3. Roll mixture into small balls and refrigerate for 30 minutes before serving.

Nutrition Information (per ball, based on 12 servings):
- Calories: 100
- Protein: 3g

- Carbohydrates: 13g
- Fat: 5g
- Fiber: 3g
- Sugar: 9g
- Portion Size: 1 ball

Peach and Berry Crumble

Ingredients:
- 2 cups peaches, sliced
- 1 cup mixed berries
- 1/2 cup oats
- 1/4 cup almond flour
- 2 tablespoons honey
- 1/4 cup coconut oil

Instructions:
1. Preheat oven to 350°F (175°C).
2. In a baking dish, combine peaches and berries.
3. In a bowl, mix oats, almond flour, honey, and melted coconut oil.
4. Sprinkle the oat mixture over the fruit.
5. Bake for 30-35 minutes, or until the topping is golden brown and the fruit is bubbling.

Nutrition Information (per serving, based on 6 servings):

- Calories: 200

- Protein: 3g

- Carbohydrates: 28g

- Fat: 8g

- Fiber: 4g

- Sugar: 18g

- Portion Size: 1/6 of recipe

Banana and Oatmeal Cookies

Ingredients:

- 2 ripe bananas, mashed

- 1 cup oats

- 1/4 cup almond butter

- 1/4 cup dark chocolate chips (optional)

Instructions:

1. Preheat oven to 350°F (175°C).

2. Mix mashed bananas, oats, and almond butter in a bowl.

3. Stir in chocolate chips if using.

4. Drop spoonfuls of the mixture onto a baking sheet.

5. Bake for 10-12 minutes, or until golden brown.

Nutrition Information (per cookie, based on 12 cookies):

- Calories: 80
- Protein: 2g
- Carbohydrates: 12g
- Fat: 3g
- Fiber: 2g
- Sugar: 7g
- Portion Size: 1 cookie

Greek Yogurt Chocolate Mousse

Ingredients:

- 1 cup plain Greek yogurt
- 1/4 cup unsweetened cocoa powder
- 2 tablespoons honey
- 1 teaspoon vanilla extract

Instructions:

1. In a bowl, mix Greek yogurt, cocoa powder, honey, and vanilla extract until smooth.
2. Chill in the refrigerator for 30 minutes before serving.

Nutrition Information (per serving, based on 2 servings):

- Calories: 140
- Protein: 10g

- Carbohydrates: 18g
- Fat: 4g
- Fiber: 3g
- Sugar: 13g
- Portion Size: 1/2 of recipe

Apple Cinnamon Muffins

Ingredients:
- 1 1/2 cups whole wheat flour
- 1/2 cup rolled oats
- 1/2 cup unsweetened applesauce
- 1/2 cup honey
- 1 teaspoon cinnamon
- 1 teaspoon baking powder
- 1/2 teaspoon baking soda
- 1 egg

Instructions:
1. Preheat oven to 350°F (175°C). Line a muffin tin with paper liners.
2. In a bowl, mix flour, oats, cinnamon, baking powder, and baking soda.
3. In another bowl, whisk applesauce, honey, and egg.
4. Combine wet and dry ingredients and mix until just blended.

5. Divide batter among muffin cups and bake for 20-25 minutes.

Nutrition Information (per muffin, based on 12 muffins):

- Calories: 150
- Protein: 4g
- Carbohydrates: 25g
- Fat: 3g
- Fiber: 3g
- Sugar: 12g
- Portion Size: 1 muffin

Frozen Banana Pops

Ingredients:

- 4 bananas, peeled and sliced into rounds
- 1/2 cup dark chocolate chips
- 2 tablespoons coconut oil
- 1/4 cup crushed nuts (optional)

Instructions:

1. Melt chocolate chips and coconut oil together in a microwave or double boiler.
2. Dip banana slices in the melted chocolate and sprinkle with crushed nuts if desired.

3. Place banana slices on a parchment-lined baking sheet and freeze for 1-2 hours.

Nutrition Information (per pop, based on 12 pops):
- Calories: 80
- Protein: 1g
- Carbohydrates: 15g
- Fat: 3g
- Fiber: 2g
- Sugar: 12g
- Portion Size: 1 pop

Sweet Potato Brownies

Ingredients:
- 1 cup mashed sweet potato
- 1/2 cup almond butter
- 1/4 cup cocoa powder
- 1/4 cup honey
- 1/4 teaspoon baking soda

Instructions:
1. Preheat oven to 350°F (175°C). Line a baking dish with parchment paper.

2. In a bowl, mix mashed sweet potato, almond butter, cocoa powder, honey, and baking soda.

3. Pour mixture into the baking dish and spread evenly.

4. Bake for 25-30 minutes. Let cool before cutting into squares.

Nutrition Information (per brownie, based on 9 brownies):

- Calories: 140
- Protein: 4g
- Carbohydrates: 20g
- Fat: 6g
- Fiber: 3g
- Sugar: 12g
- Portion Size: 1 brownie

Berry Sorbet

Ingredients:

- 2 cups mixed berries (strawberries, blueberries, raspberries)
- 1/4 cup honey or maple syrup
- 1 tablespoon lemon juice

Instructions:

1. Blend berries, honey, and lemon juice until smooth

2. Pour the mixture into a shallow dish and freeze for 2-3 hours, stirring occasionally to break up ice crystals.

3. Once firm, scoop into bowls and serve.

Nutrition Information (per serving, based on 4 servings):

- Calories: 110
- Protein: 1g
- Carbohydrates: 28g
- Fat: 0g
- Fiber: 5g
- Sugar: 23g
- Portion Size: 1/4 of recipe

Healthy Pumpkin Pie

Ingredients:

- 1 cup canned pumpkin
- 1/4 cup honey
- 2 large eggs
- 1/2 cup almond milk
- 1 teaspoon cinnamon
- 1/2 teaspoon nutmeg
- 1/4 teaspoon ginger
- 1/2 teaspoon vanilla extract
- 1 pre-made whole grain pie crust

Instructions:

1. Preheat oven to 350°F (175°C).

2. In a bowl, mix pumpkin, honey, eggs, almond milk, cinnamon, nutmeg, ginger, and vanilla extract until smooth.

3. Pour the mixture into the pie crust.

4. Bake for 45-50 minutes, or until the filling is set.

5. Allow to cool before serving.

Nutrition Information (per slice, based on 8 slices):

- Calories: 160
- Protein: 4g
- Carbohydrates: 24g
- Fat: 6g
- Fiber: 3g
- Sugar: 15g
- Portion Size: 1 slice

Oatmeal Raisin Cookies

Ingredients:

- 1 cup rolled oats
- 1/2 cup whole wheat flour
- 1/2 cup raisins
- 1/4 cup coconut oil
- 1/4 cup honey

- 1/2 teaspoon cinnamon
- 1/2 teaspoon baking soda
- 1 egg

Instructions:
1. Preheat oven to 350°F (175°C). Line a baking sheet with parchment paper.
2. In a bowl, mix oats, flour, raisins, cinnamon, and baking soda.
3. In another bowl, whisk together coconut oil, honey, and egg.
4. Combine wet and dry ingredients and mix until just blended.
5. Drop spoonfuls of dough onto the baking sheet and bake for 10-12 minutes.

Nutrition Information (per cookie, based on 12 cookies):
- Calories: 90
- Protein: 2g
- Carbohydrates: 14g
- Fat: 4g
- Fiber: 2g
- Sugar: 8g
- Portion Size: 1 cookie

No-Bake Energy Bites

Ingredients:

- 1 cup rolled oats

- 1/2 cup almond butter

- 1/4 cup honey

- 1/4 cup dark chocolate chips

- 1/4 cup chia seeds

Instructions:
1. In a bowl, mix all ingredients until well combined.
2. Roll the mixture into small balls and refrigerate for at least 30 minutes before serving.

Nutrition Information (per bite, based on 12 bites):

- Calories: 110

- Protein: 3g

- Carbohydrates: 14g

- Fat: 6g

- Fiber: 2g

- Sugar: 8g

- Portion Size: 1 bite

Fruit Salad with Mint

Ingredients:

- 1 cup strawberries, sliced
- 1 cup blueberries
- 1 cup kiwi, peeled and chopped
- 1 cup pineapple, chopped
- 2 tablespoons fresh mint leaves, chopped
- 1 tablespoon honey (optional)

Instructions:

1. In a large bowl, combine all fruit and gently toss.
2. Add mint leaves and honey if desired, and toss again.
3. Serve immediately or chill in the refrigerator for up to 1 hour.

Nutrition Information (per serving, based on 4 servings):

- Calories: 90
- Protein: 1g
- Carbohydrates: 23g
- Fat: 0g
- Fiber: 3g
- Sugar: 19g
- Portion Size: 1/4 of recipe

Chapter 7: Smoothies

Smoothies are a delightful and nutritious way to start your day or enjoy a refreshing snack. They're not only versatile but also packed with essential vitamins and minerals. This chapter explores fifteen unique smoothie recipes that are perfect for anyone looking to enhance their diet with flavorful and healthful options.

Berry Banana Smoothie

Ingredients:

- 1 banana
- 1 cup mixed berries (strawberries, blueberries, raspberries)
- 1/2 cup Greek yogurt
- 1/2 cup almond milk
- 1 tablespoon honey (optional)

Instructions:

1. Combine banana, mixed berries, Greek yogurt, and almond milk in a blender.
2. Blend until smooth. Adjust sweetness with honey if desired.
3. Pour into a glass and serve immediately.

Nutrition Information (per serving):

- Calories: 250

- Protein: 8g

- Carbohydrates: 45g

- Fat: 4g

- Fiber: 6g

- Sugar: 30g

- Portion Size: 1 glass (12 oz)

Spinach and Pineapple Smoothie

Ingredients:

- 1 cup fresh spinach

- 1 cup pineapple chunks

- 1/2 cup Greek yogurt

- 1/2 cup coconut water

- 1 tablespoon chia seeds

Instructions:

1. Add spinach, pineapple chunks, Greek yogurt, and coconut water to a blender.

2. Blend until smooth, then stir in chia seeds.

3. Serve chilled.

Nutrition Information (per serving):

- Calories: 210

- Protein: 7g

- Carbohydrates: 35g

- Fat: 2g

- Fiber: 5g

- Sugar: 30g

- Portion Size: 1 glass (12 oz)

Mango and Greek Yogurt Smoothie

Ingredients:

- 1 cup mango chunks

- 1/2 cup Greek yogurt

- 1/2 cup orange juice

- 1 tablespoon honey

- Ice cubes

Instructions:

1. Blend mango chunks, Greek yogurt, orange juice, and honey until smooth.

2. Add ice cubes for a thicker texture if desired.

3. Serve immediately.

Nutrition Information (per serving):

- Calories: 240

- Protein: 8g

- Carbohydrates: 40g

- Fat: 2g

- Fiber: 4g

- Sugar: 35g

- Portion Size: 1 glass (12 oz)

Apple Cinnamon Smoothie

Ingredients:

- 1 apple, peeled and cored

- 1/2 teaspoon ground cinnamon

- 1/2 cup Greek yogurt

- 1/2 cup almond milk

- 1 tablespoon flaxseeds

Instructions:

1. Blend apple, cinnamon, Greek yogurt, and almond milk until smooth.

2. Add flaxseeds and blend for a few more seconds.

3. Pour into a glass and enjoy.

Nutrition Information (per serving):

- Calories: 220

- Protein: 7g

- Carbohydrates: 34g

- Fat: 4g

- Fiber: 5g

- Sugar: 25g

- Portion Size: 1 glass (12 oz)

Strawberry and Kiwi Smoothie

Ingredients:

- 1 cup strawberries

- 2 kiwis, peeled

- 1/2 cup Greek yogurt

- 1/2 cup apple juice

- 1 tablespoon honey (optional)

Instructions:

1. Combine strawberries, kiwis, Greek yogurt, and apple juice in a blender.
2. Blend until smooth. Sweeten with honey if needed.
3. Serve immediately.

Nutrition Information (per serving):

- Calories: 230

- Protein: 8g

- Carbohydrates: 40g

- Fat: 2g

- Fiber: 6g

- Sugar: 30g

- Portion Size: 1 glass (12 oz)

Peach and Spinach Smoothie

Ingredients:

- 1 cup peach slices

- 1 cup fresh spinach

- 1/2 cup Greek yogurt

- 1/2 cup almond milk

- 1 tablespoon chia seeds

Instructions:

1. Add peaches, spinach, Greek yogurt, and almond milk to a blender.
2. Blend until smooth, then stir in chia seeds.
3. Serve chilled.

Nutrition Information (per serving):

- Calories: 200

- Protein: 7g

- Carbohydrates: 35g

- Fat: 2g

- Fiber: 5g

- Sugar: 25g

- Portion Size: 1 glass (12 oz)

Avocado and Banana Smoothie

Ingredients:

- 1/2 avocado

- 1 banana

- 1/2 cup Greek yogurt

- 1/2 cup almond milk

- 1 tablespoon honey

Instructions:

1. Blend avocado, banana, Greek yogurt, and almond milk until smooth.

2. Add honey and blend again.

3. Pour into a glass and enjoy.

Nutrition Information (per serving):

- Calories: 260

- Protein: 8g

- Carbohydrates: 35g

- Fat: 10g

- Fiber: 6g

- Sugar: 30g

- Portion Size: 1 glass (12 oz)

Green Smoothie with Kale and Pineapple

Ingredients:

- 1 cup kale leaves

- 1 cup pineapple chunks

- 1/2 cup Greek yogurt

- 1/2 cup coconut water

- 1 tablespoon flaxseeds

Instructions:

1. Blend kale, pineapple chunks, Greek yogurt, and coconut water until smooth.
2. Add flaxseeds and blend briefly.
3. Serve immediately.

Nutrition Information (per serving):

- Calories: 210

- Protein: 7g

- Carbohydrates: 35g

- Fat: 3g

- Fiber: 6g

- Sugar: 30g

- Portion Size: 1 glass (12 oz)

Chocolate Almond Smoothie

Ingredients:

- 1 banana

- 2 tablespoons cocoa powder

- 1/2 cup almond milk

- 1/4 cup almonds

- 1 tablespoon honey

Instructions:

1. Blend banana, cocoa powder, almond milk, and almonds until smooth.
2. Sweeten with honey if desired.
3. Serve chilled.

Nutrition Information (per serving):
- Calories: 290
- Protein: 8g
- Carbohydrates: 40g
- Fat: 12g
- Fiber: 6g
- Sugar: 30g
- Portion Size: 1 glass (12 oz)

Orange and Carrot Smoothie

Ingredients:
- 1 orange, peeled
- 1 cup carrots, chopped
- 1/2 cup Greek yogurt
- 1/2 cup apple juice
- 1 tablespoon honey (optional)

Instructions:
1. Blend orange, carrots, Greek yogurt, and apple juice until smooth.
2. Add honey for sweetness if desired.
3. Serve immediately.

Nutrition Information (per serving):
- Calories: 210

- Protein: 7g
- Carbohydrates: 35g
- Fat: 2g
- Fiber: 5g
- Sugar: 30g
- Portion Size: 1 glass (12 oz)

Blueberry and Chia Smoothie

Ingredients:
- 1 cup blueberries
- 1/2 cup Greek yogurt
- 1/2 cup almond milk
- 1 tablespoon chia seeds
- 1 tablespoon honey

Instructions:
1. Blend blueberries, Greek yogurt, and almond milk until smooth.
2. Stir in chia seeds and blend briefly.
3. Serve chilled.

Nutrition Information (per serving):
- Calories: 220
- Protein: 8g
- Carbohydrates: 35g

- Fat: 4g
- Fiber: 7g
- Sugar: 25g
- Portion Size: 1 glass (12 oz)

Tropical Fruit Smoothie

Ingredients:
- 1 cup mango chunks
- 1/2 cup pineapple chunks
- 1/2 cup Greek yogurt
- 1/2 cup coconut water
- 1 tablespoon honey (optional)

Instructions:
1. Blend mango chunks, pineapple chunks, Greek yogurt, and coconut water until smooth.
2. Sweeten with honey if desired.
3. Serve immediately.

Nutrition Information (per serving):
- Calories: 230
- Protein: 7g
- Carbohydrates: 38g
- Fat: 2g

- Fiber: 5g
- Sugar: 30g
- Portion Size: 1 glass (12 oz)

Strawberry-Banana Spinach Smoothie

Ingredients:
- 1 banana
- 1 cup strawberries
- 1 cup fresh spinach
- 1/2 cup Greek yogurt
- 1/2 cup almond milk

Instructions:

1. Blend banana, strawberries, spinach, Greek yogurt, and almond milk until smooth.
2. Pour into a glass and serve immediately.

Nutrition Information (per serving):
- Calories: 220
- Protein: 8g
- Carbohydrates: 35g
- Fat: 2g
- Fiber: 6g
- Sugar: 25g

- Portion Size: 1 glass (12 oz)

Green Apple and Celery Smoothie

Ingredients:

- 1 green apple, cored and sliced
- 2 celery stalks, chopped
- 1/2 cup Greek yogurt
- 1/2 cup almond milk
- 1 tablespoon flaxseeds

Instructions:

1. Blend green apple, celery, Greek yogurt, and almond milk until smooth.
2. Add flaxseeds and blend briefly.
3. Serve chilled.

Nutrition Information (per serving):

- Calories: 200
- Protein: 7g
- Carbohydrates: 35g
- Fat: 2g
- Fiber: 6g
- Sugar: 20g
- Portion Size: 1 glass (12 oz)

Berry and Yogurt Smoothie

Ingredients:

- 1 cup mixed berries (strawberries, blueberries, raspberries)
- 1/2 cup Greek yogurt
- 1/2 cup almond milk
- 1 tablespoon honey (optional)
- Ice cubes

Instructions:

1. Combine mixed berries, Greek yogurt, and almond milk in a blender.
2. Blend until smooth. Add honey for extra sweetness if desired.
3. Serve with ice cubes for a chilled treat.

Nutrition Information (per serving):

- Calories: 220
- Protein: 8g
- Carbohydrates: 35g
- Fat: 3g
- Fiber: 5g
- Sugar: 25g
- Portion Size: 1 glass (12 oz)

Conclusion

As we conclude our journey through the "Pre-Diabetes Cookbook for Kids," it's essential to reflect on the key principles and takeaways from the recipes and meal plans provided. This chapter serves not just as a wrap-up, but as a reminder of the importance of integrating healthy eating habits into daily life for children facing pre-diabetes.

Throughout this cookbook, we have emphasized a balanced approach to nutrition, combining the right amount of carbohydrates, proteins, and fats to support optimal health. Each recipe was selected with care to ensure that it not only meets dietary needs but also appeals to younger tastes and preferences. We've explored a variety of meals that are both nutritious and enjoyable, demonstrating that managing pre-diabetes doesn't mean sacrificing flavor or fun.

One of the most important lessons is the value of consistency. Establishing and maintaining a routine that includes wholesome, low-glycemic foods can make a significant difference in managing pre-diabetes. The 30-day meal plan was designed to offer a range of options, ensuring that kids don't feel deprived or bored with their diet. By providing a diverse selection of meals and snacks, we aim to keep children engaged and enthusiastic about their food choices.

As we close this chapter, remember that managing pre-diabetes is a continuous journey. The strategies and recipes provided here are intended to be adaptable and scalable according to individual preferences and needs. The goal is to build a sustainable lifestyle that promotes long-term health and well-being.

Thank you for allowing this cookbook to be a part of your journey. May it inspire and support you as you continue to navigate the path to managing pre-diabetes with confidence and care.

Made in the USA
Las Vegas, NV
13 September 2024